Chapter 1: Understanding Influenza

What is Influenza?

Influenza, commonly known as the flu, is a contagious respiratory illness caused by influenza viruses. These viruses primarily infect the nose, throat, and sometimes the lungs, leading to a range of symptoms that can vary in severity. Most individuals experience symptoms such as fever, cough, sore throat, body aches, headaches, chills, and fatigue. In some cases, particularly among vulnerable populations such as young children, the elderly, and individuals with pre-existing health conditions, influenza can lead to severe complications, including pneumonia, hospitalization, and even death.

Influenza viruses are categorized into four main types: A, B, C, and D. Types A and B are responsible for the seasonal flu epidemics that occur annually, while type C usually causes milder respiratory symptoms and is not associated with epidemics. Type D primarily affects cattle and is not known to infect humans. Influenza A viruses are further classified into subtypes based on two proteins on their surface: hemagglutinin (H) and neuraminidase (N). This classification system is crucial for understanding the potential for new strains to emerge and cause widespread outbreaks.

The influenza virus is highly transmissible, spreading mainly through respiratory droplets when an infected person coughs or sneezes. It can also spread by touching surfaces contaminated with the virus and then touching the face. This ease of transmission contributes to the rapid spread of influenza during seasonal outbreaks, typically occurring in the fall and winter months. Public health authorities monitor influenza activity and provide recommendations to mitigate its spread, including vaccination campaigns and public awareness initiatives about hygiene practices.

Vaccination remains the most effective method for preventing influenza infection and its complications. The formulation of the influenza vaccine is updated annually to match circulating strains, as

1

the virus is known for its ability to mutate and evolve. In addition to the standard flu vaccine, antiviral medications may be prescribed to treat influenza, particularly in high-risk patients. These medications can help reduce the duration and severity of illness if administered early in the course of the infection.

Understanding the dynamics of influenza is vital for effective outbreak management and prevention strategies. Historical pandemics, such as the 1918 Spanish flu and the H1N1 outbreak in 2009, illustrate the potential impact of influenza on public health. Continuous research into influenza virus evolution, vaccine development, and treatment options is essential for preparing for and responding to seasonal outbreaks and potential pandemics. Awareness of influenza's risks, transmission methods, and prevention strategies empowers patients to take proactive steps in safeguarding their health and that of their communities.

Types of Influenza Viruses

Influenza viruses are categorized into four main types: A, B, C, and D. Each type has distinct characteristics and implications for human health. Influenza A viruses are the most common cause of seasonal epidemics and pandemics. They can infect both humans and animals, leading to significant genetic variability. This type is further divided into subtypes based on two key surface proteins: hemagglutinin (H) and neuraminidase (N). The ability of Influenza A viruses to undergo antigenic shift and drift contributes to their potential to cause widespread outbreaks.

Influenza B viruses primarily circulate among humans and are responsible for seasonal flu outbreaks. Unlike Influenza A, which can infect a variety of animal species, Influenza B is more stable and does not exhibit the same level of genetic reassortment. Influenza B is categorized into two lineages: B/Yamagata and B/Victoria. Although less common than Influenza A, it can still lead to severe illness, particularly in vulnerable populations such as the elderly and those with underlying health conditions.

Influenza C viruses typically cause mild respiratory illness and are not associated with epidemics. They are less understood than the other types but are generally not a public health concern. Influenza D viruses primarily affect cattle and are not known to infect humans. As research continues, understanding the differences among these types is crucial for developing effective vaccines and treatments.

The implications of these different influenza types extend to public health strategies and vaccine development. Seasonal influenza vaccines are designed to protect against the most prevalent strains of Influenza A and B, tailored each year based on surveillance data. The variability of Influenza A poses challenges for vaccine formulation, necessitating ongoing monitoring and adjustments to ensure effectiveness. Additionally, antiviral treatments are generally more effective against specific strains, highlighting the importance of identifying the type of virus causing an outbreak.

Understanding the various types of influenza viruses is essential for effective outbreak management and prevention strategies. Public health campaigns often focus on promoting vaccination and awareness of influenza transmission, particularly in high-risk groups. As new strains emerge, continuous education and research are vital to mitigate the impact of influenza on communities, especially considering the potential for co-morbidities and severe complications in at-risk populations. By remaining informed about the types of influenza viruses, patients can better understand their health options and the importance of prevention measures.

Symptoms and Diagnosis

Symptoms of influenza can vary from mild to severe and typically manifest suddenly, often within one to two days after exposure to the virus. Common symptoms include a high fever, chills, cough, sore throat, runny or stuffy nose, muscle or body aches, headaches, and fatigue. Some individuals may also experience gastrointestinal symptoms, such as nausea, vomiting, or diarrhea, though these are more common in children than adults. Recognizing these symptoms early is critical, as it can lead to timely medical intervention, which may reduce the severity of the illness and prevent complications.

Diagnosing influenza generally begins with a thorough medical history and physical examination. Healthcare providers will assess the presence of classic symptoms and potential exposure to the virus. In many cases, diagnosis can be made based solely on clinical presentation, especially during peak flu season when the virus is prevalent. However, laboratory testing can confirm the diagnosis, particularly in atypical cases or for individuals at high risk of complications. Rapid influenza diagnostic tests (RIDTs) can produce results within minutes, while more sensitive tests, such as PCR (polymerase chain reaction), may take longer but provide a more accurate identification of the viral strain.

In addition to the clinical symptoms and testing methods, understanding the nuances of influenza diagnosis is essential for managing public health. During outbreaks, surveillance systems play a crucial role in tracking flu activity and informing health authorities. This data helps in identifying patterns, such as the emergence of new strains and the effectiveness of current vaccines. Public health campaigns also leverage this information to educate communities about the importance of early recognition and reporting of symptoms, which aids in outbreak management and prevention strategies.

Special considerations are necessary when diagnosing influenza in pediatric populations. Children may present with atypical symptoms or may not communicate their feelings as effectively as adults. Thus, caregivers should be vigilant for signs such as excessive irritability, lethargy, or difficulty breathing. Pediatricians may also consider the child's vaccination status and any underlying comorbidities, as these factors can influence the severity of the illness and the approach to treatment. Prompt diagnosis in children is crucial, as they are at a higher risk for developing complications such as pneumonia or bronchitis.

For individuals with existing comorbidities, such as asthma, diabetes, or cardiovascular diseases, the symptoms of influenza may be more pronounced and can lead to serious health complications. Therefore, it is vital for patients with these conditions to seek medical advice at the onset of flu-like symptoms. Healthcare providers may recommend antiviral treatments, which are most effective when administered within the first 48 hours of symptom onset. Through awareness and understanding of symptoms and prompt diagnosis, patients can take proactive steps towards managing their health during flu season and minimizing the impact of influenza on their well-being.

Chapter 2: The Importance of Vaccination

How Vaccines Work

Vaccines are crucial tools in the battle against influenza, working by stimulating the immune system to recognize and combat the virus. When a vaccine is administered, it introduces a harmless component of the virus, often in the form of inactivated virus or specific viral proteins, into the body. This exposure prompts the immune system to respond as if it were encountering the actual virus. The immune system produces antibodies, which are proteins specifically designed to fight off the virus if the body is exposed to it in the future. This process of building immunity can take several weeks, which is why it is important to get vaccinated before the onset of flu season.

The effectiveness of influenza vaccines can vary from year to year and among different populations. Each year, health officials monitor circulating strains of the virus to determine which strains are most likely to be prevalent during the upcoming flu season. Vaccines are formulated based on this data, aiming to provide the best possible protection. Among the different types of influenza vaccines available, some target three strains (trivalent vaccines), while others target four strains (quadrivalent vaccines). This adaptability is essential for addressing the evolving nature of the influenza virus, which can change rapidly.

In addition to individual protection, vaccination plays a vital role in community health. When a significant portion of the population is vaccinated, herd immunity is achieved, which helps protect those who are unable to receive vaccines, such as infants or individuals with certain medical conditions. This collective immunity slows the spread of the virus, reducing the likelihood of outbreaks. Public health campaigns often emphasize the importance of vaccination not only for personal health but also for the well-being of the community, particularly in vulnerable populations such as the elderly and those with comorbidities.

Understanding how vaccines work is particularly important for parents of pediatric patients. Children are at a higher risk for severe complications from influenza, making vaccination a crucial part of their healthcare. Pediatric formulations of the influenza vaccine are available, and guidelines recommend that children receive their annual vaccine, starting at six months of age. Parents should be aware of the recommended vaccination schedule and understand the importance of adhering to it, as timely vaccination can significantly reduce the risk of flu-related hospitalizations and complications.

Finally, while vaccines are effective, they are not the only line of defense against influenza. Antiviral medications can also play a critical role in managing the virus once someone is infected. These treatments work best when administered early in the illness and can help reduce the severity and duration of symptoms. In conjunction with vaccination, antiviral treatments enhance overall influenza management strategies, especially during outbreaks. By understanding both the preventive and therapeutic measures available, patients can better navigate the complexities of influenza and protect their health and the health of those around them.

Development of Influenza Vaccines

The development of influenza vaccines has undergone significant evolution since the first vaccines were introduced in the 1940s. Initially, these vaccines were created using killed viruses, which provided limited immunity and required annual updates to account for the rapidly changing influenza strains. Over the decades, advancements in technology and research have led to more effective vaccine formulations, including live attenuated and recombinant vaccines. This ongoing evolution is crucial for enhancing public health responses to seasonal outbreaks and potential pandemics, as the effectiveness of vaccines directly correlates with their ability to match circulating virus strains.

In recent years, the process of vaccine development has become more sophisticated, utilizing innovative techniques such as reverse genetics and cell-based production methods. Reverse genetics allows scientists to manipulate viral genes in a laboratory setting, creating vaccines that can elicit stronger immune responses. Cell-based vaccines, grown in mammalian cells rather than eggs, can be produced more rapidly and are less susceptible to the limitations posed by egg supply and viral mutations. These advancements not only improve the speed of vaccine production but also enhance the overall safety and effectiveness of the vaccines available to the public.

As influenza viruses mutate frequently, the World Health Organization plays a critical role in determining the strains that will be included in the seasonal vaccine. This decision is based on global surveillance data, which monitors circulating strains and their potential impact on public health. Consequently, patients should be aware that the composition of the vaccine may change each year, making it essential to receive the most current vaccination to ensure optimal protection. Public health campaigns emphasize the importance of annual vaccination as part of a comprehensive strategy to minimize the risk of influenza outbreaks and protect vulnerable populations, including children, the elderly, and those with underlying health conditions.

The development of antiviral treatments has also complemented vaccine efforts in managing influenza outbreaks. Antivirals can reduce the severity and duration of influenza symptoms when administered early in the course of the illness. Patients, especially those at higher risk due to comorbidities, should be informed about the availability of these treatments as an added layer of protection alongside vaccination. Education about the combined benefits of vaccination and antiviral medications is crucial in enhancing patient outcomes during influenza seasons.

Ultimately, the ongoing research and development of influenza vaccines reflect the dynamic nature of public health and the commitment to safeguarding communities. Patients are encouraged to stay informed about the latest influenza trends, vaccine recommendations, and outbreak management strategies. By understanding the importance of vaccination in preventing influenza transmission and its associated complications, individuals can take proactive steps to protect themselves and their loved ones, contributing to a healthier society overall.

Types of Influenza Vaccines

Influenza vaccines are essential tools in the fight against seasonal flu and pandemic strains, and understanding the different types can help patients make informed decisions about their health. The primary categories of influenza vaccines include inactivated, live attenuated, and recombinant vaccines. Inactivated vaccines are the most commonly administered and contain virus particles that have been killed, ensuring they cannot cause disease. These vaccines are typically injected and are suitable for most age groups, including those with underlying health conditions.

Live attenuated influenza vaccines (LAIV) are another option, consisting of weakened forms of the virus that are still capable of eliciting an immune response without causing illness. LAIV is administered as a nasal spray and is generally recommended for healthy individuals aged two to forty-nine. However, caution is advised for individuals with certain comorbidities, as the live virus, although weakened, might pose risks. Understanding the eligibility for LAIV is vital for patients, especially those considering vaccination for their children or themselves.

Recombinant influenza vaccines represent a newer innovation in vaccine technology. These vaccines are created using genetic engineering to produce a portion of the influenza virus, which helps stimulate an immune response without using the live virus. Recombinant vaccines are particularly beneficial for individuals with egg allergies, as they are produced without the need for egg-based culture systems typically used in traditional vaccine production. This advancement expands the options available to patients who may have had previous concerns about receiving the flu shot.

Additionally, there are quadrivalent vaccines, which protect against four different strains of the influenza virus, including two A strains and two B strains. This broader coverage is crucial as influenza viruses can mutate and change from year to year. By receiving a quadrivalent vaccine, patients increase their chances of being protected against the most prevalent strains circulating during a given flu season. Public health campaigns often highlight the importance of annual vaccination with the latest formulations to keep up with evolving influenza trends.

Understanding the types of influenza vaccines helps patients navigate their options and encourages proactive health measures. With the potential for influenza outbreaks and the associated risks, particularly for vulnerable populations such as children and those with comorbidities, timely vaccination becomes even more critical. By staying informed about vaccine types and their benefits, patients can contribute to their own health and the broader community's efforts in influenza prevention and control.

Vaccine Efficacy and Safety

Vaccine efficacy and safety are critical components in the fight against influenza, particularly given the virus's ability to mutate and cause seasonal outbreaks. The effectiveness of a vaccine is determined by its ability to evoke an immune response that protects the individual from contracting the virus or reduces the severity of illness if infection occurs. Influenza vaccines are designed to match the circulating strains of the virus, which is why annual vaccination is necessary. The efficacy of these vaccines can vary from season to season, depending on factors such as the match between the vaccine strains and the circulating strains, the age and health of the population being vaccinated, and the presence of coexisting medical conditions.

The safety of influenza vaccines is thoroughly evaluated through rigorous clinical trials before they are approved for public use. Regulatory agencies, such as the U.S. Food and Drug Administration

(FDA) and the World Health Organization (WHO), monitor vaccine safety continuously. Common side effects are usually mild and may include soreness at the injection site, low-grade fever, and muscle aches. Serious adverse reactions are rare, and the benefits of vaccination—such as protection against severe illness, hospitalization, and death—far outweigh the risks. Public health organizations actively promote vaccination as a key strategy for reducing the overall impact of influenza in communities.

In pediatric populations, the efficacy of the influenza vaccine is particularly important, as children are often at a higher risk of severe illness due to influenza. The immune response in children can differ from adults, which is why specific formulations, such as the nasal spray vaccine, are available for younger patients. Studies have shown that pediatric vaccines can significantly reduce the incidence of influenza-related complications, including hospitalization. Vaccination not only protects children but also helps to reduce the spread of the virus within schools and households, contributing to community immunity.

Understanding seasonal influenza trends and statistics is essential for appreciating the role of vaccines in public health. Epidemiological data provide insight into the prevalence of different influenza strains, the effectiveness of vaccines in various demographics, and the overall impact of vaccination campaigns. When high vaccination rates are achieved, the incidence of influenza outbreaks declines, leading to fewer hospitalizations and deaths. Public health campaigns often emphasize the importance of vaccination, especially for high-risk groups, such as the elderly, pregnant women, and individuals with chronic health conditions.

In the context of influenza transmission and infection control, vaccination serves as a primary line of defense. The vaccine not only protects individuals but also contributes to herd immunity, which is vital for safeguarding vulnerable populations. When a significant portion of the community is vaccinated, the spread of the virus is hindered, reducing the likelihood of outbreaks. Historical pandemics highlight the importance of vaccination strategies in managing influenza. By learning from past experiences and continuously improving vaccine development and distribution, public health officials can better prepare for seasonal influenza and potential pandemics, ensuring that safety and efficacy remain at the forefront of influenza prevention efforts.

Chapter 3: Influenza Outbreak Management

Recognizing an Outbreak

Recognizing an outbreak of influenza is crucial for both individual and community health. Influenza outbreaks can occur seasonally, but they may also arise unexpectedly due to factors such as changes in the virus, population immunity, and environmental conditions. Awareness of the signs and symptoms of influenza, alongside knowledge of how outbreaks manifest in the community, can empower patients to take proactive steps in seeking care and preventing further spread. Typical symptoms include fever, cough, sore throat, body aches, and fatigue, which often appear abruptly. Understanding these symptoms in the context of a community outbreak is essential in distinguishing influenza from other respiratory illnesses.

Monitoring seasonal trends and statistics is vital for recognizing potential outbreaks. Public health agencies frequently release data on influenza activity, including the percentage of positive tests, hospitalizations, and mortality rates. Patients should familiarize themselves with local health department resources, as these provide updates on the current influenza season and any unusual spikes in cases. Additionally, awareness of historical patterns can offer insights into when outbreaks are most likely to occur, ultimately enabling patients to prepare for potential illness during peak times.

Influenza transmission occurs through respiratory droplets when an infected person coughs, sneezes, or talks. Recognizing the mechanisms of transmission can help patients identify high-risk situations, such as crowded places or close contact with infected individuals. Furthermore, understanding that influenza viruses can survive on surfaces for a limited time underscores the importance of hygiene practices, such as regular handwashing and disinfecting shared spaces. Awareness of these transmission dynamics can inform patients on how to protect themselves and their loved ones during an outbreak.

Public health campaigns play a critical role in educating the community about influenza prevention. These initiatives often promote vaccination, encourage proper respiratory hygiene, and provide guidance on recognizing outbreak signs. Patients should actively engage with these campaigns, as they offer valuable information on the timing and availability of vaccines, as well as updates on ongoing outbreaks. Participation in these campaigns can enhance community resilience and reduce the overall impact of influenza on public health.

For patients with comorbidities, recognizing an outbreak is even more critical, as they are at higher risk for severe complications. Conditions such as asthma, diabetes, and heart disease can exacerbate the effects of influenza, making awareness and early intervention essential. Patients with these conditions should monitor health advisories closely and consult healthcare providers regarding vaccination and antiviral treatments. By staying informed and taking preventive measures, patients can better navigate the complexities of influenza outbreaks and safeguard their health and well-being.

Public Health Response

Public health response to influenza encompasses a range of strategies aimed at mitigating the impact of seasonal outbreaks and potential pandemics. This multifaceted approach involves surveillance, vaccination campaigns, antiviral treatment protocols, and public education initiatives. By understanding these components, patients can better navigate their health choices during influenza season and contribute to community efforts aimed at reducing the spread of the virus.

Surveillance is crucial for monitoring influenza trends and identifying potential outbreaks. Public health agencies collect and analyze data on influenza cases, hospitalizations, and deaths. This information helps to track seasonal patterns, recognize atypical strains, and assess the effectiveness of vaccines. Patients can play a role in this process by reporting symptoms and seeking medical attention when needed. Awareness of local influenza activity can empower individuals to take preventive measures, such as receiving vaccinations or practicing good hygiene.

Vaccination remains the cornerstone of public health response to influenza. Annual flu vaccines are designed to protect against the most prevalent strains of the virus. Public health campaigns often focus on increasing vaccination rates among high-risk populations, including children, the elderly, and individuals with comorbidities. Patients should understand the importance of timely vaccination, not only for their own health but also for the broader community. Herd immunity can significantly reduce the spread of influenza, making it vital for as many people as possible to be vaccinated each season.

In addition to vaccination, antiviral treatments are an essential aspect of managing influenza outbreaks. Medications such as oseltamivir and zanamivir can reduce the severity and duration of symptoms if taken early in the course of the illness. Public health responses often include guidelines for the use of these treatments, particularly for vulnerable populations. Patients should be informed about the availability of antiviral medications and the importance of early intervention in improving outcomes, especially for those with underlying health conditions.

Public health campaigns play a pivotal role in educating patients about influenza prevention and transmission control. These initiatives often promote key practices such as hand hygiene, respiratory etiquette, and staying home when ill. Understanding how influenza spreads can help patients take proactive steps to protect themselves and others. Additionally, recognizing the historical context of influenza pandemics can enhance awareness of the virus's potential impact. By fostering a culture of prevention and awareness, public health responses aim to create a more informed patient population capable of navigating the complexities of influenza effectively.

Community Preparedness

Community preparedness plays a crucial role in managing influenza outbreaks and minimizing their impact on public health. Effective community preparedness involves establishing robust systems for surveillance, communication, and response strategies that engage various stakeholders, including healthcare providers, local government, and the public. Understanding the dynamics of influenza transmission is essential for communities to implement appropriate measures to reduce the risk of infection and protect vulnerable populations, particularly those with comorbidities or in pediatric age groups.

One of the key components of community preparedness is education and awareness. Public health campaigns aimed at informing the community about the importance of vaccination, recognizing symptoms, and knowing when to seek medical help can significantly enhance community resilience. These campaigns often utilize multiple platforms, including social media, community workshops, and collaboration with local schools and organizations. By fostering an informed population, communities can ensure higher vaccination rates and better adherence to public health recommendations during influenza season.

Surveillance is another critical aspect of community preparedness. Monitoring influenza trends and statistics enables public health officials to identify outbreaks early and allocate resources effectively. Communities should establish local surveillance systems that report cases to health authorities, allowing for timely interventions. This data can inform decisions about when to implement specific public health measures, such as closing schools, canceling large gatherings, or enforcing infection control protocols in healthcare settings. Engaging the public in reporting influenza-like illnesses can also enhance surveillance efforts.

Effective communication during an influenza outbreak is vital for managing public perception and compliance with health guidelines.

Communities should develop clear protocols for disseminating timely and accurate information regarding the status of influenza activity, vaccine availability, and treatment options. Utilizing trusted local figures and healthcare professionals can help convey messages effectively and build public trust. Transparency in communication fosters a cooperative environment where individuals feel empowered to take precautions, such as practicing good hygiene and staying home when ill.

Lastly, community preparedness must include plans for healthcare resource management. During an influenza outbreak, healthcare systems can be overwhelmed, making it essential for communities to have strategies in place for allocating resources, including antiviral treatments and hospital beds. Collaboration between local healthcare providers, public health officials, and emergency services ensures that communities are ready to respond effectively to surges in demand. By prioritizing community preparedness, individuals can contribute to a collective effort to mitigate the effects of influenza and protect public health.

Chapter 4: Antiviral Treatments for Influenza

Overview of Antiviral Medications

Antiviral medications play a crucial role in the management of influenza, particularly in reducing the severity and duration of the illness. These medications are designed to inhibit the replication of the influenza virus, providing patients with a better chance of recovery, especially when administered early in the course of the infection. The most commonly prescribed antiviral drugs for influenza include oseltamivir (Tamiflu), zanamivir (Relenza), and peramivir (Rapivab). Each of these medications works by targeting specific proteins on the virus, effectively limiting its ability to spread within the body.

Oseltamivir is an oral medication that is often preferred due to its ease of administration and broad availability. It is effective against both influenza A and B viruses and is typically recommended for individuals who exhibit symptoms within the first 48 hours of onset. This time frame is critical, as the effectiveness of antiviral treatment diminishes significantly when initiated later in the course of the illness. Zanamivir, administered via inhalation, is another option, particularly for patients who may not tolerate oral medications or for those with specific respiratory conditions. Peramivir, an intravenous formulation, is used primarily in hospitalized patients who require immediate treatment.

The use of antiviral medications is particularly important in high-risk populations, including children, the elderly, and individuals with underlying health conditions such as asthma or diabetes. In these groups, influenza can lead to severe complications, making timely intervention with antivirals essential. Clinical studies have shown that early administration of these medications can reduce the risk of hospitalization and improve outcomes in patients with comorbidities. Additionally, for pediatric populations, careful consideration of dosing and potential side effects is necessary, as children may respond differently to antiviral treatments compared to adults.

While antivirals are an important tool in the fight against influenza, they are not a substitute for vaccination. The influenza vaccine remains the primary method of prevention and is recommended for everyone over the age of six months. Vaccination not only helps protect individuals from contracting influenza but also reduces the overall spread of the virus within communities. Public health campaigns emphasize the importance of vaccination in conjunction with antiviral medications to mitigate the impact of seasonal influenza outbreaks.

Continued research and development of antiviral medications are vital as influenza viruses evolve and new strains emerge. Understanding the trends and statistics associated with seasonal influenza can inform public health strategies and improve treatment protocols. As the landscape of influenza changes, staying informed about available antiviral options and their appropriate use can empower patients and their families to make informed decisions regarding their health and wellness during flu season.

When to Seek Treatment

Recognizing the appropriate time to seek treatment for influenza is crucial for effective management and recovery. Influenza symptoms can range from mild to severe, and understanding the severity of your symptoms can help determine whether medical intervention is necessary. If you experience common symptoms such as fever, cough, sore throat, body aches, chills, fatigue, or headache, it is important to monitor their intensity and duration. If symptoms persist for more than a few days or worsen, it may be time to consult a healthcare professional.

Certain populations are at higher risk for complications from influenza, including young children, elderly individuals, pregnant women, and those with underlying health conditions such as asthma, diabetes, or heart disease. If you belong to one of these high-risk categories or live with someone who does, seeking treatment early can be pivotal. Antiviral medications can be most effective when initiated within the first 48 hours of symptom onset, potentially reducing the severity and duration of the illness.

In addition to individual symptoms and risk factors, pay attention to warning signs that indicate a more severe illness. Difficulty breathing, chest pain, sudden dizziness, confusion, or persistent vomiting are serious symptoms that require immediate medical attention. These signs may suggest complications such as pneumonia or other respiratory issues, which can arise from influenza infections and necessitate urgent care.

Seasonal trends can also inform your decision to seek treatment. During peak influenza season, healthcare systems may be under strain due to higher patient volumes. If you suspect you have influenza during an outbreak, prompt action is advisable to ensure proper diagnosis and treatment. Public health campaigns often emphasize the importance of early intervention, which can also contribute to community health by preventing the spread of the virus.

Finally, staying informed about influenza vaccination and local outbreak statistics can guide your approach to treatment. Vaccination remains a key preventive measure, but breakthrough infections can still occur. Understanding the current influenza strains circulating in your area can help assess your risk and the need for treatment. Always consult with a healthcare provider if you have questions about your symptoms or the appropriateness of antiviral medications based on current influenza trends.

Managing Side Effects

Managing side effects associated with influenza vaccines and antiviral treatments is crucial for maximizing patient comfort and adherence to recommended health measures. Understanding these side effects can empower patients to make informed decisions about their health. Common side effects of influenza vaccines include soreness at the injection site, mild fever, fatigue, and muscle aches. These reactions are generally mild and resolve on their own within a few days. Recognizing that these symptoms are normal responses to vaccination can help alleviate concerns and encourage patients to follow through with immunization.

For those undergoing antiviral treatment for influenza, side effects may vary depending on the specific medication prescribed. Common antiviral drugs, such as oseltamivir and zanamivir, can cause gastrointestinal disturbances, headaches, and, in rare cases, neuropsychiatric symptoms. It is essential for patients to communicate any adverse reactions to their healthcare provider, as this information can guide adjustments to treatment plans and enhance overall management of influenza. Monitoring side effects closely is vital, particularly in pediatric populations, where reactions may differ from those in adults.

Patients with pre-existing comorbidities must be particularly vigilant about managing side effects. Conditions such as asthma, diabetes, or heart disease can complicate the clinical picture when experiencing both influenza symptoms and treatment side effects. It is advisable for patients to maintain open lines of communication with their healthcare providers regarding any underlying conditions and to report increased severity of side effects. Tailoring flu management strategies to accommodate existing health issues can lead to better outcomes and a smoother recovery process.

Public health campaigns often emphasize the importance of vaccination and early treatment, but they also play a role in educating patients about managing side effects. Informing the community about what to expect post-vaccination or during antiviral treatment can enhance public confidence in these interventions. Campaigns that highlight resources for managing side effects, such as hot compresses for injection site pain or hydration strategies for gastrointestinal issues, can further support patients in navigating their treatment journeys.

Finally, understanding the historical context of influenza pandemics can provide perspective on the importance of managing side effects effectively. Past outbreaks have demonstrated that the benefits of vaccination and antiviral treatment far outweigh the risks of side effects. As influenza continues to evolve, staying informed about the latest research and recommendations can empower patients to take proactive steps in their care. By managing side effects effectively, individuals can contribute to broader public health goals, ensuring that vaccination rates remain high and that antiviral treatments are utilized effectively in the face of seasonal influenza.

Chapter 5: Special Considerations for Pediatric Populations

Influenza Symptoms in Children

Influenza symptoms in children can vary significantly from those in adults, and understanding these differences is crucial for parents and caregivers. Children often exhibit classic flu symptoms such as fever, chills, and body aches. However, they may also experience gastrointestinal symptoms like nausea, vomiting, or diarrhea, which are less common in adults. A child suffering from influenza may become unusually fatigued and irritable, and they may show a decreased interest in play or normal activities. Recognizing these signs early can help in seeking timely medical assistance and reducing the risk of complications.

Fever is one of the most prominent symptoms of influenza in children and can often reach high temperatures, sometimes above 104°F. This elevated fever can lead to discomfort and lethargy, making it essential for parents to monitor their child's temperature regularly. Alongside fever, cough and sore throat are typical respiratory symptoms that can exacerbate the overall feeling of illness. These respiratory issues may lead to labored breathing or a persistent cough, which can be distressing for both the child and the parents. Understanding the range of respiratory symptoms can assist caregivers in determining when to seek medical advice.

Children with influenza may also experience muscle and joint pain, which can make simple movements painful and further contribute to their overall discomfort. These symptoms can be particularly challenging for younger children who may not articulate their feelings effectively. It is important for caregivers to observe behavioral changes, as children might express their discomfort through irritability or changes in sleeping patterns. Additionally, children with underlying health conditions, such as asthma or diabetes, may experience exacerbated symptoms, necessitating closer monitoring and possibly more aggressive treatment strategies.

Complications from influenza can arise, especially in pediatric populations. Symptoms such as difficulty breathing, persistent high fever, or severe dehydration warrant immediate medical attention. Influenza can lead to secondary bacterial infections like pneumonia, which pose serious risks to children's health. Parents should be educated about these potential complications and the importance of following up with healthcare providers if their child's symptoms worsen or do not improve within a few days. Being aware of these risks can empower parents to act swiftly and appropriately.

In light of these symptoms and potential complications, vaccination against influenza is a critical preventive measure for children. The influenza vaccine can significantly reduce the severity of symptoms and the risk of hospitalization. Public health campaigns emphasize the importance of annual vaccinations, particularly for young children, who are at a higher risk of severe illness. By understanding the symptoms of influenza and the importance of vaccination, parents can take proactive steps to protect their children and contribute to broader public health efforts aimed at managing influenza outbreaks effectively.

Vaccination for Children

Vaccination plays a crucial role in protecting children from influenza, a virus that poses significant health risks to this vulnerable population. The influenza vaccine is designed to stimulate the immune system, preparing it to recognize and combat the virus effectively. Annual vaccination is recommended for children aged six months and older, as the virus can mutate and circulate in different strains each year. This variability underscores the importance of receiving the vaccine annually to ensure optimal protection against the most prevalent strains.

The development of the influenza vaccine has undergone significant advancements since its inception. Modern vaccines are tailored to include the most current strains of the virus, based on surveillance data collected by health organizations worldwide. These vaccines are available in various forms, including inactivated virus vaccines and live attenuated vaccines, catering to different age groups and health conditions. Pediatric populations are particularly targeted in vaccination campaigns due to their heightened susceptibility to severe influenza complications, such as pneumonia and hospitalization.

During influenza outbreaks, public health campaigns emphasize the importance of vaccination for children. These initiatives often aim to educate parents about the benefits of immunization, not only for the individual child but also for the broader community. High vaccination rates among children can contribute to herd immunity, reducing the overall transmission of the virus. Public health authorities also collaborate with schools and childcare centers to facilitate vaccination programs, making it more accessible for families to participate.

Despite the proven efficacy of the influenza vaccine, some parents may still have concerns about its safety and side effects. Research consistently indicates that the benefits of vaccination far outweigh the risks, with mild side effects such as soreness at the injection site or low-grade fever being common. Serious adverse reactions are exceedingly rare. Healthcare professionals play a vital role in addressing these concerns, providing evidence-based information that helps parents make informed decisions regarding their children's health.

In conclusion, vaccination remains a cornerstone of influenza prevention in pediatric populations. By ensuring that children receive their annual flu shots, parents not only protect their children from potentially severe illness but also contribute to the overall health and safety of their communities. Continued efforts in education and outreach are essential to improve vaccination rates and combat the impact of influenza, particularly during seasonal epidemics and potential pandemics.

Treatment Options for Pediatric Patients

Treatment options for pediatric patients diagnosed with influenza are crucial for ensuring their recovery and minimizing complications. In children, the presentation of influenza can vary widely, and understanding the appropriate therapeutic interventions is essential for parents and caregivers. The primary goal of treatment is to alleviate symptoms, prevent complications, and reduce the duration of illness. Pediatric patients may benefit from a combination of antiviral medications, supportive care, and preventive measures.

Antiviral medications play a significant role in the treatment of influenza in children. Oseltamivir (Tamiflu) and zanamivir (Relenza) are commonly prescribed antiviral agents that can shorten the duration of symptoms and may decrease the risk of severe complications when administered early in the course of the illness. The effectiveness of these medications is most pronounced when given within the first 48 hours of symptom onset. For pediatric patients, the dosage and duration of antiviral therapy are carefully determined based on age, weight, and overall health status, ensuring optimal treatment outcomes.

In addition to antiviral treatments, supportive care is vital for managing pediatric influenza. This includes ensuring proper hydration, encouraging rest, and administering fever-reducing medications such as acetaminophen or ibuprofen, as recommended by a healthcare provider. Parents should monitor their child's symptoms closely, watching for signs of dehydration or difficulty breathing, which may necessitate further medical attention. Creating a comfortable environment and providing age-appropriate activities can also help children cope with the illness while they recover.

Prevention remains a cornerstone of managing influenza in pediatric populations. Annual influenza vaccinations are highly recommended for children aged six months and older. Vaccination not only protects the individual child but also contributes to community immunity, reducing the overall spread of the virus. Public health campaigns emphasize the importance of vaccination, particularly for children with underlying health conditions that may increase their risk for influenza complications. Parents are encouraged to consult with healthcare providers about the best vaccination strategies for their children.

Lastly, it is important for parents to be aware of the broader context of influenza management and its implications for pediatric health. Historical data indicates that children are disproportionately affected by influenza-related complications, especially during peak outbreak seasons. Understanding seasonal trends and adhering to public health guidelines can significantly reduce the risk of transmission and promote effective infection control within homes and communities. By staying informed and proactive, parents can navigate the complexities of influenza treatment and prevention for their pediatric patients effectively.

Chapter 6: Seasonal Influenza Trends and Statistics

Annual Patterns of Influenza

Annual patterns of influenza are characterized by predictable seasonal trends, which can significantly impact public health and individual well-being. Influenza typically exhibits a seasonal cycle, peaking during the colder months of the year. In temperate regions, this peak generally occurs between December and February, while in tropical areas, influenza can circulate year-round with distinct peaks at different times. Understanding these patterns is crucial for patients as it helps in recognizing the best times for vaccination and awareness of potential outbreaks.

The influenza virus is known for its ability to mutate, leading to variations in its strains from year to year. This antigenic drift and shift contribute to the annual variability observed in influenza cases. Health authorities, including the World Health Organization, closely monitor these changes to update vaccine formulations accordingly. For patients, this means that receiving a vaccine each year is necessary to ensure protection against the most prevalent strains circulating during the flu season. Staying informed about vaccine updates and recommendations can aid in personal preventive measures.

Influenza outbreaks can occur sporadically and are often influenced by various factors, including environmental conditions, population density, and vaccination rates. The spread of the virus is facilitated by close contact among individuals, making public health campaigns essential in mitigating the impact of influenza. Community awareness initiatives emphasize the importance of vaccination, hand hygiene, and respiratory etiquette. Patients should recognize their role in these campaigns, as individual actions contribute to broader public health efforts and can significantly reduce transmission rates.

Treatment options for influenza have evolved, with antiviral medications available to reduce the severity and duration of symptoms. Timely administration of antiviral drugs is critical, particularly for high-risk populations such as young children, the elderly, and individuals with underlying health conditions. Patients should seek medical advice promptly if they exhibit flu-like symptoms, as early intervention can lead to better outcomes. Understanding the availability and effectiveness of these treatments can empower patients to take proactive steps in managing their health during influenza season.

Lastly, the interplay between influenza and comorbidities is a significant concern, as individuals with pre-existing health conditions are at greater risk for severe illness. Conditions such as asthma, diabetes, and heart disease can complicate influenza infections, necessitating a more vigilant approach to prevention and treatment. Public health messaging should focus on educating patients about the increased risks associated with comorbidities and the importance of vaccination and regular health check-ups. By staying informed and proactive, patients can navigate the challenges of influenza effectively and protect their health and the health of those around them.

Tracking Influenza Activity

Tracking influenza activity is essential for understanding the patterns of this virus and preparing for its seasonal impact. Surveillance systems collect data on influenza cases and monitor trends, allowing health officials to identify when and where outbreaks occur. This information is crucial for patients, as it informs public health campaigns and vaccine distribution efforts. By understanding the current influenza activity in their area, patients can take proactive measures to protect themselves and their families, especially during peak seasons.

Public health organizations, such as the Centers for Disease Control and Prevention (CDC) and the World Health Organization (WHO), play vital roles in tracking influenza. They use a combination of laboratory testing, outpatient visits, and hospitalizations to monitor the spread of the virus. Reports are generated weekly during flu season, providing updates on circulating strains and geographic spread. Patients can utilize these reports to gauge the severity of influenza in their communities and adjust their preventive behaviors accordingly, such as getting vaccinated or practicing better hygiene.

Influenza tracking also encompasses monitoring vaccine effectiveness and adaptability in response to circulating strains. As the virus evolves, seasonal vaccines are updated to ensure they provide adequate protection. Tracking the activity of influenza viruses and their mutations helps researchers refine vaccine formulations. Patients should be aware of the importance of annual vaccinations as part of their strategy to combat influenza, especially since some groups, such as children and individuals with comorbidities, may face greater risks.

Antiviral treatments are another critical component of influenza management. Tracking influenza activity aids in determining the prevalence of antiviral-resistant strains, which can affect treatment options. For patients, understanding the landscape of treatment availability and effectiveness is vital. If they contract influenza, they should discuss with their healthcare providers the most appropriate antiviral medications, particularly those that are effective against the current circulating strains.

Finally, historical data on influenza outbreaks can provide insights into future trends and preparedness strategies. By examining past pandemics and seasonal variations, public health officials can develop comprehensive response plans. Patients benefit from being informed about historical patterns, as they can understand the potential risks and the importance of vaccination and symptom management. Awareness of influenza transmission and infection control measures can empower patients to take an active role in protecting themselves and their communities from the virus.

Impact of Influenza Seasonality

The impact of influenza seasonality is a critical aspect of understanding how this virus behaves and affects populations each year. Influenza typically exhibits a seasonal pattern, with outbreaks occurring more frequently during the colder months in temperate regions. This seasonality is attributed to several factors, including environmental conditions that favor virus survival and transmission, as well as human behaviors that change with the seasons. As temperatures drop and people congregate indoors, the likelihood of influenza transmission increases, leading to higher infection rates. Understanding these patterns can help patients prepare and take preventive measures during peak seasons.

During each influenza season, health authorities monitor trends and statistics to track the virus's spread and inform public health campaigns. These campaigns often emphasize the importance of vaccination, particularly before the onset of the season. Vaccines are developed annually based on predictions of which influenza strains are likely to circulate, and timely vaccination can significantly reduce the incidence of illness and complications. Patients who understand the significance of getting vaccinated prior to the season can contribute to herd immunity, protecting not only themselves but also vulnerable populations such as the elderly and those with comorbidities.

Influenza's seasonality also influences the management of outbreaks. Public health officials utilize surveillance data to implement early intervention strategies, such as community awareness campaigns and vaccination drives. When an outbreak occurs, they may recommend additional measures such as antiviral treatments to mitigate the spread and severity of the illness. Patients should be aware that antiviral medications can be most effective when administered early in the course of the infection, underscoring the importance of recognizing symptoms and seeking medical advice promptly during peak influenza periods.

In pediatric populations, the impact of influenza seasonality can be particularly pronounced. Children are often more susceptible to the virus due to their developing immune systems, and they can be significant vectors for transmission within communities. Seasonal trends suggest that influenza can lead to increased hospitalizations among children, especially those with underlying health conditions. Parents should ensure their children receive the influenza vaccine annually and stay informed about the signs of influenza, as early detection can lead to better outcomes.

Finally, understanding the historical context of influenza evolution and pandemics provides insight into current trends and prevention strategies. Past pandemics have shaped public health responses and vaccine development, emphasizing the need for ongoing research and preparedness. By recognizing the cyclical nature of influenza infections and the factors that influence their seasonality, patients can become proactive participants in their own health management and contribute to broader community efforts to reduce the impact of influenza each year.

Chapter 7: Public Health Campaigns for Influenza Prevention

Key Messaging and Strategies

Key messaging and strategies are essential components in effectively communicating the importance of influenza awareness, prevention, and treatment. Patients must understand the significance of staying informed about influenza, especially during peak seasons when outbreaks are common. Clear messaging can provide clarity on the nature of the virus, its transmission, and the critical role vaccinations play in safeguarding individual and community health. Community outreach and educational campaigns should focus on dispelling myths related to the influenza vaccine and emphasizing its safety and efficacy, particularly among vulnerable populations.

Influenza vaccine development is a dynamic and ongoing process, requiring constant adaptation to emerging strains of the virus. Messaging should highlight the importance of receiving the vaccine annually, as the virus continually evolves. Patients should be encouraged to consult with healthcare providers about the latest developments in vaccine technology and recommendations. Clear communication regarding vaccine availability, administration sites, and the timing of vaccinations can significantly increase participation rates, ultimately reducing the incidence of influenza.

Effective outbreak management relies on timely and precise communication strategies. Patients need to be informed about the signs and symptoms of influenza, as well as the appropriate steps to take if they suspect they have contracted the virus. Public health campaigns should provide guidance on when to seek medical assistance, reinforcing the importance of early intervention. Additionally, patients should be made aware of the antiviral treatments available and their effectiveness in reducing the severity and duration of influenza, particularly in high-risk groups such as the elderly and those with underlying health conditions.

Influenza has a unique impact on pediatric populations, necessitating tailored messaging strategies for families. Parents should receive clear information about the increased risk of complications in children and the importance of vaccination. Educational materials should address common concerns, such as the safety of vaccines for children and the potential side effects. Strategies that involve schools and childcare centers in disseminating information can further enhance awareness and encourage proactive health behaviors among families.

Lastly, understanding the relationship between influenza and comorbidities is vital for effective patient messaging. Individuals with chronic health conditions, such as asthma, diabetes, or heart disease, are at greater risk for severe influenza-related complications. Messaging should emphasize the importance of preventive measures for these populations, including vaccination and infection control practices. Public health campaigns should also prioritize educating patients about the historical context of influenza pandemics and the evolution of the virus, fostering a greater appreciation for ongoing preventive measures and the importance of community health initiatives.

Community Outreach Programs

Community outreach programs play a vital role in the prevention and management of influenza, particularly in fostering awareness and promoting vaccination among diverse populations. These programs are designed to reach individuals who may have limited access to healthcare information or services, thereby addressing disparities in health literacy and vaccination rates. By engaging with communities through educational initiatives, health fairs, and informational workshops, these programs aim to empower individuals with the knowledge they need to protect themselves and their families from influenza.

One of the primary objectives of community outreach is to increase awareness about the importance of influenza vaccination. Public health campaigns often emphasize the safety and efficacy of vaccines, addressing common misconceptions and fears surrounding their use. Through targeted messaging and community engagement, these programs can encourage individuals, particularly those in pediatric populations and high-risk groups, to seek vaccination. This proactive approach not only helps to reduce the incidence of the virus but also contributes to herd immunity, protecting those who are unable to be vaccinated due to medical reasons.

In addition to vaccination promotion, community outreach programs provide essential information on influenza transmission and infection control measures. By educating the public about how influenza spreads and the importance of practicing good hygiene, such as handwashing and respiratory etiquette, these programs help to mitigate the risk of outbreaks. Educational materials, workshops, and interactive sessions can be tailored to meet the needs of specific demographics, including families, schools, and workplaces, ensuring that the information is relevant and accessible to all community members.

Furthermore, these outreach efforts often extend to individuals with comorbidities, who may face increased risks during influenza seasons. Tailored interventions for these populations can include providing information on how to manage their conditions in conjunction with influenza prevention strategies. By addressing the unique challenges faced by individuals with chronic health issues, community outreach programs can enhance their understanding of the need for timely vaccination and the role of antiviral treatments in managing influenza symptoms.

Ultimately, the success of community outreach programs lies in their ability to foster collaboration between healthcare providers, local organizations, and community members. By leveraging resources and expertise, these programs can create a supportive environment that encourages vaccination and promotes health literacy. As influenza trends continue to evolve, ongoing community engagement will be crucial in adapting strategies to meet the changing needs of populations, ensuring that everyone has the tools to navigate influenza effectively.

Evaluating Campaign Effectiveness

Evaluating the effectiveness of campaigns aimed at preventing and managing influenza is crucial for ensuring that public health strategies are successful. Campaign effectiveness can be assessed through a variety of metrics, including vaccination rates, public awareness, behavior change, and overall health outcomes. For patients, understanding how these evaluations take place can provide insights into the importance of participating in influenza prevention efforts, such as getting vaccinated and adhering to public health guidelines.

One key metric in evaluating campaign effectiveness is the vaccination rate among specific populations. Public health campaigns often target areas with the highest incidence of influenza or vulnerable groups such as children, the elderly, and individuals with comorbidities. By monitoring vaccination coverage, health officials can determine whether outreach efforts are reaching the intended audience and whether those individuals are following through with vaccination. High vaccination rates generally indicate a successful campaign, while low rates can highlight the need for improved messaging or access to vaccines.

Public awareness and knowledge about influenza prevention also play a significant role in evaluating campaign effectiveness. Surveys and studies can gauge how well the public understands the risks associated with influenza and the importance of vaccination. Effective campaigns should not only inform individuals about the availability of vaccines but also address common misconceptions about influenza and its transmission. As patients become more informed, they are likely to adopt preventive measures, which can decrease the incidence of influenza outbreaks in the community.

Behavior change is another critical aspect to consider. Evaluating whether patients and communities have adopted recommended practices, such as proper hand hygiene, staying home when sick, and advocating for vaccination, can provide insights into campaign success. Changes in behavior can be tracked through various methods, including observational studies and self-reported surveys. Successful campaigns often lead to increased community participation in preventive actions, thereby reducing the spread of influenza.

Finally, assessing health outcomes related to influenza, such as hospitalization rates and complications, can provide a comprehensive view of campaign effectiveness. By analyzing data pre- and post-campaign implementation, public health officials can determine the impact of their efforts on overall community health. For patients, understanding these outcomes can reinforce the importance of their participation in influenza prevention strategies, highlighting how individual actions contribute to the broader public health landscape. Evaluating campaign effectiveness ultimately helps refine future initiatives, ensuring that they are well-targeted and impactful in reducing the burden of influenza.

Chapter 8: Influenza and Comorbidities

High-Risk Groups

High-risk groups for influenza include individuals who are more susceptible to severe illness and complications from the virus. Understanding these groups is crucial for effective prevention and management strategies. Among the most vulnerable are young children, particularly those under the age of five, and elderly adults aged 65 and older. These populations often have weaker immune systems, making it difficult for them to fight off infections. Additionally, pre-existing health conditions such as asthma, diabetes, and heart disease significantly increase the risk of severe influenza-related complications.

Pregnant women also fall into the high-risk category, as their altered immune system can make them more susceptible to infections. Influenza during pregnancy can lead to serious health issues for both the mother and the developing fetus, including preterm labor and low birth weight. The Centers for Disease Control and Prevention recommends that pregnant women receive the influenza vaccine to protect themselves and their babies, highlighting the importance of vaccination in this group.

Healthcare workers and caregivers of high-risk individuals are another critical high-risk group. Due to their close contact with patients and vulnerable populations, they are more likely to be exposed to the virus and can inadvertently spread it to those they care for. Vaccination is essential for these individuals to prevent outbreaks in healthcare settings and to protect the patients they serve. Public health campaigns often emphasize the importance of flu shots for healthcare professionals to mitigate the risk of transmission.

Individuals with immunocompromising conditions, whether due to diseases like HIV/AIDS, cancer, or treatments such as chemotherapy, are also at increased risk of severe influenza. Their weakened immune systems struggle to fend off infections, making it vital for them to receive the influenza vaccine and adhere to strict infection control measures. Understanding the implications of influenza for these individuals can help tailor public health messaging and resources effectively.

Lastly, the presence of comorbidities, such as chronic respiratory diseases or obesity, further elevates the risk for severe influenza outcomes. Managing these conditions effectively and ensuring that individuals within these high-risk groups are vaccinated annually can significantly reduce the incidence of influenza-related complications. Public health initiatives aimed at educating these populations about their risks and promoting vaccination and preventive measures can play a pivotal role in reducing influenza's impact on society.

Managing Comorbid Conditions

Managing comorbid conditions is crucial for patients at risk of influenza complications. Comorbidities, such as diabetes, chronic respiratory diseases, and cardiovascular issues, can significantly increase the severity of influenza infections. Understanding how these conditions interact with influenza is essential for effective prevention and management strategies. Patients with comorbid conditions should be particularly vigilant during flu season and engage in proactive health measures to mitigate risks associated with influenza.

One of the primary strategies for patients with comorbid conditions is to maintain regular communication with healthcare providers. This includes discussing the appropriate timing for influenza vaccination, which can provide critical protection against the virus. Vaccination is especially important for individuals with underlying health issues, as they are more susceptible to severe outcomes. Healthcare providers can offer tailored advice on vaccination schedules, potential side effects, and the need for booster shots in some cases. Patients should also be encouraged to report any changes in their health status that might impact their risk for influenza.

In addition to vaccination, managing comorbid conditions effectively is vital. This includes adhering to prescribed treatments and medications, monitoring symptoms, and maintaining a healthy lifestyle. Regular exercise, a balanced diet, and adequate sleep can enhance overall health and boost the immune system's ability to fight infections. Patients should work closely with their healthcare teams to develop individualized plans that address both their comorbidities and influenza prevention strategies. Effective management of chronic conditions can lead to better outcomes if influenza infection occurs.

Patients should also be educated about the signs of influenza and the importance of early intervention. Recognizing early symptoms can facilitate prompt treatment, which is especially critical for those with comorbidities. Antiviral treatments may be prescribed to lessen the severity of influenza and reduce the duration of illness. Patients should understand the importance of seeking medical attention at the first sign of flu-like symptoms, as timely antiviral therapy can significantly improve their health trajectory.

Lastly, public health campaigns play a significant role in raising awareness about the interaction between influenza and comorbid conditions. These campaigns can provide valuable information regarding the importance of vaccination, symptom recognition, and preventive measures. By fostering a better understanding of how comorbidities affect influenza risks, patients can become proactive participants in their health management. Engaging in community resources and educational programs can empower patients to navigate their health challenges more effectively, ultimately leading to better outcomes during flu seasons.

Preventive Strategies for At-Risk Patients

Preventive strategies for at-risk patients play a crucial role in managing influenza effectively, especially considering the potential severity of the illness in vulnerable populations. At-risk individuals often include young children, the elderly, pregnant women, and those with underlying health conditions such as asthma, diabetes, or heart disease. Understanding these strategies not only empowers patients but also enhances community health by minimizing the spread of the virus.

Vaccination remains the cornerstone of prevention for at-risk populations. The seasonal influenza vaccine is updated annually to match circulating strains, providing the best chance of protection. It is particularly essential for those with comorbidities, as their immune systems may not respond as robustly to the virus. Additionally, public health campaigns emphasize the importance of annual vaccination, often targeting high-risk groups through community outreach and educational programs. Patients should consult their healthcare providers about getting vaccinated and any specific recommendations based on their health status.

In addition to vaccination, practicing good hygiene is vital for preventing influenza transmission. Regular handwashing with soap and water, or using hand sanitizer when soap is unavailable, can significantly reduce the risk of contracting or spreading the virus. Patients should also be encouraged to avoid close contact with individuals exhibiting flu-like symptoms and to maintain a clean environment by disinfecting frequently touched surfaces. These simple yet effective practices can help safeguard not only at-risk patients but the broader community as well.

Antiviral treatments also play a critical role in managing influenza, particularly for those already at risk. Early intervention with antiviral medications can reduce the severity and duration of the illness when administered within the first 48 hours of symptom onset. Healthcare providers should educate patients on recognizing early symptoms and the importance of seeking prompt medical attention. For individuals with chronic health issues, having a proactive plan in place, including access to antiviral medications, can be life-saving.

Finally, understanding seasonal trends and statistics surrounding influenza can help at-risk patients make informed decisions about their health. Awareness of peak influenza seasons allows individuals to take extra precautions during high-risk periods. Public health organizations often publish data on influenza activity, outbreaks, and vaccination rates, which patients should monitor. By staying informed and engaged with preventive strategies, at-risk patients can better navigate their health during flu season, ultimately leading to improved health outcomes and reduced transmission within the community.

Chapter 9: Transmission and Infection Control

How Influenza Spreads

Influenza primarily spreads through respiratory droplets when an infected person coughs, sneezes, or talks. These droplets can travel short distances—typically around six feet—before settling on surfaces or being inhaled by individuals nearby. Close contact is a significant factor in transmission; therefore, crowded places, especially during the flu season, become hotspots for the virus. Understanding this mode of transmission is crucial for patients, as it emphasizes the importance of maintaining physical distance and practicing good respiratory hygiene to mitigate the risks associated with influenza.

In addition to respiratory droplets, influenza can also spread via surfaces contaminated with the virus. When an infected person touches their mouth or nose and then touches a surface, the virus can survive on that surface for several hours. If another person touches the contaminated surface and then touches their face, they can introduce the virus into their body. This indirect transmission highlights the necessity of frequent handwashing and the use of hand sanitizers, particularly in public spaces where the risk of touching contaminated surfaces is higher.

Seasonal trends in influenza transmission reveal patterns that can help patients prepare and protect themselves. Influenza viruses tend to circulate more widely during the fall and winter months, leading to seasonal outbreaks. Public health campaigns often aim to increase awareness and encourage vaccination during these peak periods. Patients should stay informed about local flu activity through health department reports and be proactive in getting vaccinated ahead of the flu season to boost their immunity.

Certain populations are at higher risk for severe influenza-related complications, such as young children, the elderly, and individuals with comorbidities like asthma, diabetes, or heart disease. These groups not only experience higher transmission rates but also face greater health risks if infected. Understanding the vulnerability associated with these conditions can motivate patients to take preventive actions seriously. It is essential for patients with comorbidities to consult healthcare providers for tailored advice on vaccination and antiviral treatments.

Infection control measures are critical in both healthcare settings and the community to limit the spread of influenza. Strategies such as mask-wearing, especially in crowded indoor environments, can significantly reduce transmission rates. Awareness of the symptoms of influenza, along with a prompt response to any signs of infection, can also help in early diagnosis and treatment. By understanding how influenza spreads, patients can adopt appropriate measures to protect themselves and their loved ones, contributing to overall community health and safety during flu seasons.

Preventive Measures in Daily Life

Preventive measures in daily life are essential in reducing the spread of influenza and protecting both individual and community health. The first line of defense against influenza is vaccination. Annual flu shots are recommended for everyone aged six months and older, particularly those in high-risk categories, such as young children, the elderly, and individuals with chronic health conditions. Vaccination not only lowers the risk of contracting the virus but also helps mitigate the severity of the disease if infection occurs. Staying informed about the timing and availability of vaccines is critical; optimal vaccination typically takes place in the early fall, just before the flu season peaks.

In addition to vaccination, practicing good hygiene is vital in preventing the transmission of influenza. Regular handwashing with soap and water for at least 20 seconds is one of the most effective ways to eliminate germs. When soap and water are not available, alcohol-based hand sanitizers can be a suitable alternative. Avoiding close contact with individuals who show symptoms of influenza, such as coughing and sneezing, is equally important. Covering the mouth and nose with a tissue or the elbow when sneezing or coughing can help prevent the spread of respiratory droplets, which are a primary mode of influenza transmission.

Maintaining a healthy lifestyle can significantly bolster the immune system and improve overall resilience against influenza. A balanced diet rich in fruits, vegetables, whole grains, and lean proteins provides essential nutrients that support immune function. Regular physical activity, adequate sleep, and stress management also play critical roles in enhancing immunity. Patients should be encouraged to establish routines that incorporate these healthy habits into their daily lives, as they not only help in preventing influenza but also contribute to overall well-being.

In environments prone to outbreaks, such as schools, workplaces, and healthcare settings, implementing infection control measures is crucial. This may include regular cleaning and disinfection of frequently touched surfaces, ensuring proper ventilation in indoor spaces, and encouraging sick individuals to stay home. Public health campaigns often emphasize the importance of these measures, particularly during peak flu season, to raise awareness and encourage collective action. For families, discussing these preventive strategies can foster a culture of health and safety, especially among children who may not fully understand the implications of influenza.

Finally, staying informed about influenza trends and statistics can empower patients to take proactive steps in their health management. Understanding the patterns of seasonal influenza and recognizing the signs and symptoms of the virus can lead to earlier intervention and treatment. Patients should be encouraged to engage with reliable sources of information, such as public health agencies and healthcare providers, to remain updated on recommendations for prevention and treatment. By taking these preventive measures in daily life, individuals can play a significant role in curbing the spread of influenza and protecting their communities.

Infection Control in Healthcare Settings

Infection control in healthcare settings is a cornerstone of safeguarding patients from the spread of influenza and other infectious diseases. Healthcare facilities, where vulnerable populations often seek treatment, are at heightened risk for outbreaks. The transmission of influenza viruses can occur through direct contact with infected individuals or contaminated surfaces, as well as through respiratory droplets expelled during coughing or sneezing. Understanding the mechanisms of transmission is vital for both healthcare providers and patients to implement effective preventive measures.

One of the primary strategies for infection control is the use of personal protective equipment (PPE). Healthcare workers are trained to wear masks, gloves, gowns, and eye protection when interacting with patients who exhibit influenza-like symptoms. This practice minimizes the risk of virus transmission and protects both healthcare personnel and other patients. Additionally, patients themselves are encouraged to wear masks when symptomatic, creating a barrier that helps reduce the spread of respiratory droplets in waiting rooms and treatment areas.

Another crucial aspect of infection control is the rigorous cleaning and disinfection of surfaces and equipment. High-touch areas, such as doorknobs, light switches, and examination tables, must be regularly sanitized with appropriate disinfectants known to be effective against influenza viruses. Healthcare facilities also implement environmental monitoring to ensure that infection control protocols are being followed. This vigilance is particularly important during peak flu seasons when the likelihood of outbreaks is elevated.

Vaccination remains one of the most effective tools for preventing influenza transmission in healthcare settings. Annual vaccination of healthcare workers not only protects them but also helps create herd immunity within the facility. Patients who are admitted to hospitals or outpatient clinics are often encouraged to receive the influenza vaccine, especially those in high-risk categories, such as the elderly or individuals with chronic health conditions. Public health campaigns play a vital role in promoting vaccination and educating patients about the importance of protecting themselves and their communities.

In conclusion, infection control in healthcare settings is essential for preventing influenza outbreaks and ensuring patient safety. Both healthcare providers and patients must be actively engaged in infection prevention strategies, including the use of PPE, proper sanitation practices, and vaccination efforts. By fostering a culture of vigilance and awareness, healthcare facilities can significantly reduce the risk of influenza transmission, ultimately protecting the health of all individuals within these environments.

Chapter 10: Historical Pandemics and Influenza Evolution

Major Influenza Pandemics

Major influenza pandemics have profoundly shaped public health responses and vaccine development throughout history. The most notable pandemics occurred in 1918, 1957, 1968, and 2009, each marked by the rapid spread of the virus and significant mortality rates. The 1918 Spanish Flu pandemic, caused by the H1N1 virus, is often cited as the deadliest, infecting approximately one-third of the global population and resulting in an estimated 50 million deaths. This pandemic highlighted the importance of understanding viral transmission and the necessity for effective public health campaigns and interventions.

The emergence of new influenza strains often results from genetic mutations and reassortment, which can lead to pandemics. The 1957 Asian Flu and the 1968 Hong Kong Flu were both caused by H2N2 and H3N2 viruses, respectively. These outbreaks emphasized the importance of rapid surveillance and response mechanisms to manage emerging threats. Public health authorities learned that timely vaccination and antiviral treatments are crucial in controlling outbreaks and mitigating the impact of such pandemics on healthcare systems.

In recent years, the 2009 H1N1 pandemic, also known as the swine flu, demonstrated the ongoing threat of influenza viruses to global health. This outbreak was characterized by a novel strain that originated from swine and quickly spread among humans. It led to a renewed focus on vaccine development and the need for effective antiviral treatments. The swift response, including the deployment of a vaccine within months of the outbreak, showcased advancements in vaccine technology and the importance of preparedness in managing influenza pandemics.

The impact of influenza extends beyond the immediate health crisis, particularly among vulnerable populations such as children and those with comorbidities. Pediatric populations are at risk for severe complications from influenza, highlighting the need for targeted public health campaigns that emphasize vaccination for children and their caregivers. Likewise, individuals with chronic health conditions, such as asthma or diabetes, face increased risks, necessitating tailored prevention strategies that address their specific health needs.

Understanding historical pandemics informs current strategies for prevention and management of influenza. By studying the patterns of transmission and the effectiveness of past public health campaigns, health professionals can better prepare for future outbreaks. Continuous monitoring of influenza trends and statistics is essential for adapting strategies to combat seasonal flu and potential pandemics. As patients, staying informed about vaccination, antiviral treatments, and infection control measures can empower individuals to protect themselves and their communities against the threat of influenza.

Lessons Learned from History

Lessons learned from history regarding influenza provide invaluable insights for patients navigating their understanding of the disease and its prevention. Historical pandemics, such as the 1918 Spanish flu, reveal the devastating impact that influenza can have on populations. This pandemic resulted in millions of deaths worldwide, underscoring the importance of effective public health measures. By studying past outbreaks, we can better appreciate the necessity of vaccination, social distancing, and other preventive strategies that have emerged as critical tools in managing influenza today.

Vaccine development has evolved significantly over the decades, informed by lessons from previous influenza outbreaks. The rapid mutation of the influenza virus necessitates ongoing research to develop effective vaccines that can adapt to emerging strains.

Understanding the historical challenges in vaccine production helps patients appreciate the complexity of vaccination efforts. For instance, the difficulties faced during the 1976 swine flu vaccination campaign serve as a reminder of the importance of thorough testing and public communication to ensure safety and efficacy, ultimately fostering greater public trust in vaccination efforts.

Outbreak management strategies have also been shaped by historical experiences. The response to the H1N1 pandemic in 2009 highlighted the importance of timely public health interventions and the role of communication in mitigating the spread of the virus. By learning from the successes and failures of past outbreak responses, health authorities can refine their strategies, ensuring that patients are informed and prepared in the event of an influenza outbreak. This historical context empowers patients to understand their roles in outbreak management, including the importance of vaccination and adherence to public health guidelines.

Antiviral treatments for influenza have a history of development that reflects the ongoing struggle to combat the virus effectively. Lessons from previous pandemics have driven the research and approval of antiviral medications, which can significantly reduce the severity and duration of influenza when administered early. Patients should be informed about the availability of these treatments and the importance of seeking medical care promptly, especially for vulnerable populations such as children and those with comorbidities. Understanding the evolution of treatment options can encourage patients to engage proactively in their healthcare.

Lastly, the impact of influenza on pediatric populations is a critical area where historical lessons have informed current practices. Past outbreaks have shown that children are at particular risk for severe complications from influenza, leading to enhanced emphasis on vaccination and preventive measures within this demographic. Public health campaigns have increasingly targeted families with children, highlighting the necessity of vaccination and education on infection control practices. By learning from history, patients can advocate for themselves and their families, ensuring they are protected against the ongoing threat of influenza.

The Future of Influenza Research

The future of influenza research is poised to make significant advancements that will enhance our understanding of the virus, improve prevention strategies, and develop more effective treatments. As scientists continue to study the genetic variations of influenza strains, we can expect to see the emergence of more precise vaccines tailored to specific populations and circulating strains. This could be particularly beneficial in managing seasonal outbreaks, where the timely adaptation of vaccines to match circulating viruses will play a critical role in public health.

One promising area of research focuses on universal influenza vaccines, which aim to provide broader protection against multiple strains of the virus. Unlike traditional vaccines that may need to be reformulated each year, a universal vaccine could reduce the burden of annual vaccinations and improve immunity longevity. This advancement would be especially advantageous for vulnerable populations, including children and individuals with comorbidities, who are at greater risk for severe complications from influenza. Ongoing clinical trials and studies will be essential in determining the efficacy and safety of these new vaccine formulations.

In addition to vaccine development, antiviral treatments are also evolving. The future of antiviral medications for influenza looks to incorporate novel compounds and treatment regimens that may reduce the duration and severity of illness. Research is underway to identify new targets for antiviral action, which could lead to more effective drugs and the potential for combination therapies. These advancements will be vital in managing influenza outbreaks, particularly in high-risk populations and during pandemics, where timely intervention can save lives.

Public health campaigns will also play a crucial role in the future of influenza management. Increasing awareness about the importance of vaccination and preventive measures will help mitigate the impact of seasonal influenza and reduce transmission rates. As research continues to uncover trends and statistics related to seasonal influenza, public health officials can better tailor their messaging and interventions to address specific community needs. Engaging with the public through education and outreach will foster a culture of prevention that is essential for managing influenza effectively.

Finally, understanding the historical context of influenza evolution will illuminate future research directions. By examining past pandemics and the virus's adaptive mechanisms, researchers can identify patterns that may predict future outbreaks. This knowledge is invaluable in preparing for potential influenza threats and developing strategies to control transmission. As we move forward, a collaborative approach involving researchers, healthcare providers, and public health officials will be essential in shaping the future landscape of influenza research, ultimately leading to better outcomes for patients.